INTERMITTENT FASTING

DIET

The comprehensive Guide for Fast and Easy Weight Loss, Slow Aging and Improve the Quality of Life Through the Process of intermittent fasting.

11 BOOK OF 12

BY Davis Smith

Chapter 1. Effect of Intermittent Fasting on Maximal Strength in Humans

Intermittent fasting (IF) is an inexorably well-known dietary methodology utilized for weight reduction and generally wellbeing. While there is an expanding collection of proof exhibiting helpful impacts of IF on blood lipids and other wellbeing results in the overweight and corpulent, restricted information are accessible about the impact of IF in competitors. Consequently, the current examination tried to explore the impacts of an altered IF convention (for example time-limited taking care of) during opposition preparing in sound obstruction prepared guys.

INTERMITTENT FASTING

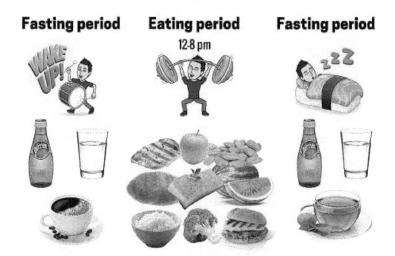

Fasting period   **Eating period**   **Fasting period**

12-8 pm

1.1 Background

Fasting, the deliberate restraint from food consumption for a predefined timeframe, is a notable practice related with numerous strict and otherworldly customs. Truth be told, this austere practice is referred to in the Old Testament, just as other antiquated messages such the Koran and the Mahabharata. In people, fasting is accomplished by ingesting practically zero food or caloric refreshments for periods that normally range from 12 hours to 3 weeks. Muslims, for instance, quick from day break until sunset during the long stretch of Ramadan, while Christians, Jews, Buddhists, and Hindus customarily quick on assigned days or periods. Fasting is unmistakable from caloric limitation (CR), in which every day caloric admission is constantly decreased by up to 40 %, however supper recurrence is kept up. As opposed to fasting, starvation is an ongoing wholesome lack that is usually mistakenly utilized as a substitute for the expression "fasting". Starvation could likewise allude to some limit types of fasting, which can bring about a hindered metabolic state and passing. In any case, starvation normally suggests persistent compulsory restraint of food, which can prompt supplement lacks and wellbeing impedance. While a drawn out time of fasting is hard to perform for the ordinary populace, an intermittent fasting (IF) convention has been appeared to deliver higher consistence. Regularly, IF is characterized by a total or fractional limitation in energy admission (somewhere in the range of 50 and 100 % limitation of absolute every day energy consumption) on 1–3 days of the week or a total limitation in energy consumption for a characterized period during the day that expands the overnight quick. The most concentrated of the above type of IF is Ramadan fasting: during the heavenly month of Ramadan, which changes as indicated by the lunar schedule, Muslims swear off eating or drinking from dawn to nightfall. The impacts of Ramadan have been broadly examined, on wellbeing results, yet in addition on practice execution. In addition, lately an emphasis on different types of IF, disconnected to strict practice, has arisen. One such structure, substitute day fasting (ADF; fasting each and every other day) is coordinated with rotating "feast days," on which there is an "not obligatory" energy admission, and "quick days" with decreased or invalid energy consumption.

A developing assortment of proof proposes that, as a rule, IF could address a helpful device for improving wellbeing in all inclusive community because of reports of improving blood lipids and glycaemic control, lessening flowing insulin, diminishing circulatory strain, diminishing provocative markers and decreasing fat mass in any event, during moderately brief lengths (8–12 weeks). These announced impacts are likely interceded through changes in metabolic pathways and cell cycles, for example, stress obstruction, lipolysis, and autophagy. One specific type of IF which has acquired extraordinary prominence through traditional press is the supposed time-confined taking care of (TRF). TRF permits subjects to burn-through not obligatory energy admission inside a characterized window of time (from

3–4 hours to 10–12 hours), which implies a fasting window of 12–21 hours of the day is utilized. A central issue concerning the IF approach is that for the most part calorie admission isn't controlled, yet the taking care of times are.

In sports, IF is concentrated chiefly in relationship with Ramadan period, while TRF has gotten mainstream among wellness experts asserting assumed consequences for support of bulk and fat misfortune. Exceptionally restricted logical data is accessible about TRF and competitors, and blended outcomes have been accounted for. We exhibited as of late that TRF didn't influence absolute body arrangement nor effect muscle cross-sectional region following two months in youthful beforehand undeveloped men performing opposition preparing, in spite of a detailed decrease in energy admission of 650 kcal each fasting day in the TRF bunch. Accordingly the point of the current examination was to research the impacts of an isoenergetic TRF convention on body piece, athletic execution, and metabolic elements during obstruction preparing in sound opposition prepared guys. We guessed that the TRF convention would prompt more prominent fat misfortune and upgrades in wellbeing related biomarkers when contrasted with a commonplace eating plan.

1.2 Methods

34 opposition prepared guys were haphazardly appointed to time-confined taking care of (TRF) or ordinary eating routine gathering (ND). TRF subjects devoured 100 % of their energy needs in an 8-hours timeframe every day, with their caloric admission isolated into three suppers burned-through at 1 p.m., 4 p.m., and 8 p.m. The leftover 16 h each 24-hours' time span made up the fasting time frame. Subjects in the ND bunch burned-through 100 % of their energy needs separated into three dinners devoured at 8 a.m., 1 p.m., and 8 p.m. Gatherings were coordinated for kilocalories burned-through and macronutrient dissemination. Subjects were tried when two months of the allocated diet and normalized opposition preparing program. Fat mass and without fat mass were evaluated by double energy x-beam absorptiometry and muscle space of the thigh and arm were estimated utilizing an anthropometric framework. Aggregate and free testosterone, insulin-like development factor 1, blood glucose, insulin, adiponectin, leptin, triiodothyronine, thyroid animating chemical, interleukin-6, interleukin-1 beta, tumor rot factor alpha, absolute cholesterol, high-thickness lipoprotein cholesterol, low-thickness lipoprotein cholesterol, and fatty oils were estimated. Seat press and

leg press maximal strength, resting energy use, and respiratory proportion were additionally tried.

Subjects

34 obstruction prepared guys were selected through promotions set in Veneto locale's exercise centers. The rules for entering the investigation were that subjects more likely than not performed obstruction preparing constantly for in any event 5 years (preparing 3–5 days/week with at any rate 3 years' involvement with split preparing schedules), be by and by occupied with customary opposition preparing at the hour of enlistment, be long lasting steroid free, and have no clinical issues that could be irritated by the examination systems.

53 subjects reacted to the promotion, however 7 were rejected for past utilization of anabolic steroids, and 12 declined investment after clarification of study's convention. In this manner, 34 subjects (age 29.21; weight 84 kg) were haphazardly appointed to a period limited taking care of gathering (TRF; n is equivalent to 17) or standard eating routine gathering (ND; n is equivalent to 17) through PC created programming. The examination staff directing result evaluations was unconscious of the task of the subjects (for example a

solitary visually impaired plan). Anthropometric gauge attributes of subjects. All members read and marked an educated assent record with the portrayal of the testing techniques endorsed by the moral advisory group, and adjusted to eat less carbs

Dietary admission was estimated by an approved 7-day food journal, which has been utilized in past investigations with competitors, and broke down by nourishing programming. Subjects were told to keep up their routine caloric admission, as estimated during the fundamental seven day stretch of the examination. During the 8-week exploratory period, TRF subjects devoured 100 % of their energy needs partitioned into three suppers burned-through at 1 p.m., 4 p.m. furthermore, 8 p.m., and abstained for the excess 16 hours each 24-hours' time frame. ND bunch ingested their caloric admission as three suppers devoured at 8 a.m., 1 p.m. furthermore, 8 p.m. This dinner timing was picked to make a fair appropriation of the three suppers during the taking care of period in the TRF convention, while the timetable for the ND bunch kept an ordinary feast dissemination (breakfast toward the beginning of the day, lunch at 1 p.m. also, supper at 8 p.m.). The conveyance of calories was 40, 25, and 35 % at 1 p.m., 4 p.m. furthermore, 8 p.m. individually for TRF, while ND subjects devoured 25, 40 and 35 % of day by day calories at 8 a.m., 1 p.m. also, 8 p.m. individually. The particular calorie conveyance was allotted by a nutritionist and depended on the revealed every day admission of each subject principles for the utilization of human subjects in research as illustrated in the flow affirmation.

ND subjects were told to devour the whole breakfast feast between 8 a.m. furthermore, 9 a.m., the whole lunch dinner between 1 p.m. what's more, 2 p.m., and the whole supper feast between 8 p.m. what's more, 9 p.m. TRF subjects were told to devour the main supper between 1 p.m. furthermore, 2 p.m., the second supper between 4 p.m. also, 5 p.m., and the third feast between 8 p.m. what's more, 9 p.m. No snacks between the suppers were permitted with the exception of 20 grams of whey proteins 30 minutes after each instructional meeting. Consistently, subjects were reached by a dietician to check the adherence to the eating routine convention. The dietician played out an organized meeting about supper timing and creation to get this data.

Training

Preparing was normalized for the two gatherings, and all subjects had at any rate 5 years of persistent opposition preparing experience before the examination. Preparing comprised of 3 week after week meetings performed on non-sequential days for about two months. All members began the trial methods in the long stretches of January or February 2014.

The obstruction preparing program comprised of 3 diverse week after week meetings (for example a split daily practice): meeting A (seat press, slant hand weight fly, biceps twist), meeting B (military press, leg press, leg expansion, leg twist), and meeting C (wide hold pull down, invert grasp pull down and rear arm muscles push down). The preparation convention included 3 arrangements of 6–8 redundancies at 85–90 % 1-RM, and reiterations were performed to disappointment (for example the failure to play out another reiteration with right execution) with 180 s of rest among sets and activities. The strategy of preparing to strong disappointment was picked on the grounds that it is quite possibly the most well-known practices for jocks, and it was a recognizable procedure for the subjects. True to form, the muscle activity speed fluctuated between subjects because of their diverse anatomical influence. In spite of the fact that there was slight variety of redundancy rhythm for each subject, the normal term of every reiteration was roughly 1.0 s for the concentric stage and 2.0 s for the unconventional stage.

The examination group straightforwardly administered all schedules to guarantee legitimate execution of the everyday practice. Every week, loads were acclimated to keep up the objective reiteration range with a compelling burden. Instructional courses were performed somewhere in the range of 4:00 and 6:00 p.m. Subjects were not permitted to perform different activities other than those remembered for the trial convention.

Measurements

Body weight was estimated to the closest 0.1 kg utilizing an electronic scale, and stature to the closest 1 cm utilizing a divider mounted compact meter. Weight file (BMI) was determined in kg. Fat mass and without fat mass were surveyed by double energy X-beam absorptiometry. Muscle territories were determined utilizing the accompanying anthropometric framework. We estimated appendage perimeters to the closest 0.001 m utilizing an anthropometric tape at the mid-arm and mid-thigh. We additionally estimated biceps, rear arm muscles, and thigh skinfolds to the closest 1 mm utilizing a caliper. All estimations were taken by a similar administrator (AP) previously and during the investigation as indicated by standard systems. Muscle regions were then determined utilizing a formerly approved programming. Cross-sectional region (CSA) estimated with has contrasted with attractive reverberation and an ICC of 0.988 and 0.968 for thigh and arm, individually.

Ventilator estimations were made by standard open-circuit calorimeter with breath-by-breath methodology. The gas examination framework was utilized: Oxygen take-up and carbon dioxide yield esteems were estimated and used to ascertain resting energy consumption (REE) and respiratory proportion (RR) utilizing the altered Weir condition. Prior to every estimation, the calorimeter was warmed by the maker's guidelines and adjusted with reference gases of known organization preceding every member.

Oxygen take-up was estimated (mL/min) and furthermore standardized to body weight (mL/kg/min), and the respiratory proportion was resolved. In the wake of resting for 15 minutes, the information were gathered for 30 minutes, and just the last 20 min were utilized to figure the respiratory gas boundaries. All tests were acted in the first part of the day somewhere in the range of 6 and 8 a.m. while the subjects were recumbent. The room was faintly lit, calm, and around 23 °C. Subjects were approached to swear off caffeine, liquor utilization and from enthusiastic active work for 24 hours preceding the estimation.

Blood analysis protocol

Blood tests taken from the vein at standard and following two months were gathered in BD containers. Tests were centrifuged (4000 RPM at 4 °C utilizing axis), and the resultant serum was aliquot and put away at short 80 °C. All examples were investigated in a similar scientific meeting for each test utilizing a similar reagent parcel. Prior to the scientific meeting, the serum tests were defrosted for the time being at 4 °C and afterward blended. Interleukin-6 (IL-6), tumor corruption factor (TNF), and interleukin-1 beta were estimated utilizing immunoassay unit. The between examine coefficient of varieties (CVs) were 3.5–6.2 and 3.2–6.3 % for IL-6, TNF and IL-1 beta separately. Insulin-like development factor 1 (IGF-1) was estimated utilizing the analyzer Liaison XL. This test is a sandwich immunoassay dependent on a disclosure, and the CV for IGF-1 was somewhere in the range of 5.6 and 9.6 %; the reference range for this test relies upon age and sex. Fasting complete cholesterol, high-thickness lipoprotein cholesterol (HDL-C), low-thickness lipoprotein cholesterol (LDL-C), and fatty oils (TG) were estimated by an enzymatic colorimetric strategy utilizing a measured. LDL-C part was determined from recipe. The between test CVs for all out cholesterol, HDL-C, and triacylglycerol focuses were 2.9, 1.8, and 2.4 %, separately. Glucose was estimated in three-fold by the glucose oxidase strategy, with a CV of 1.2 %. Leptin and adiponectin were estimated by radioimmunoassay utilizing financially accessible units (Leptin and Adiponectin); insulin was estimated with an immunoassay. The measure affectability was 1 mL, and between and intra-examine CVs were under 10, 5, and 6 % for leptin, adiponectin, and insulin, separately. Thyroid-animating chemical (TSH), free (T4) and (T3) were estimated via robotized strategies. Plasma testosterone was resolved utilizing Testosterone II performed on particular analyzer with discovery.

Tests for Strength

One redundancy most extreme (1-RM) for the leg press and the seat press practices was estimated on discrete days. Subjects executed a particular get ready for every 1-RM test by performing 5 reiterations with a weight they could typically lift multiple times. Utilizing methods portrayed somewhere else, the weight was steadily expanded until disappointment happened in both of the activities tried. The best burden lifted was viewed as the 1-RM. Recently distributed ICCs for test–retest unwavering quality for leg press and seat press 1-RM testing was 0.997 and 0.997, separately, in men, with a coefficient of variety of 0.235 for LP and 0.290 for BP. 1-RM was additionally evaluated at pattern and following 4 and two months for all preparation practices so the essential changes for conceivable strength increments could be made, consequently guaranteeing that subjects kept on preparing at an overall power of 85–90 % of their 1-RM.

Analysis of Stats

Results are introduced as mean standard deviation. The example size was acquired expecting a cooperation of a root mean square normalized impact of 0.25 with a fixed force of 80 % and an alpha danger of 5 % for the fundamental variable. Through the test, we surveyed the ordinariness. An autonomous examples test was utilized to test gauge contrasts between gatherings. The two-way rehashed measures customary ANOVA was performed (utilizing time as the inside subject factor and diet as the between-subject factor) to evaluate contrasts between bunches throughout the investigation. Additionally we received a blended model ANOVA in with the fixed variable fat mass communicated in kg as covariate versus Time increase by Diet as arbitrary factors. All distinctions were considered critical at P is equivalent to 0.05. Post-hoc investigations were performed utilizing the test. To decrease the impact of inside bunch fluctuation a trial of importance (ANCOVA) was performed. We fixed as depended variable the pre-post for each gathering and the benchmark upsides of the results were embraced as covariate; IF versus ND were expected as absolute indicators.

1.3 Results

Following two months, a critical abatement in fat mass was seen in the TRF bunch, while sans fat mass was kept up in the two gatherings. A similar pattern was noticed for arm and thigh muscle cross-sectional region. Leg press maximal strength expanded altogether, however no distinction was available between medicines. Complete testosterone and IGF-1 diminished altogether in TRF following two months while no critical contrasts were distinguished in ND. Blood glucose and insulin levels diminished fundamentally just in TRF subjects and conformingly a critical improvement of HOMA-IR was distinguished. In the TRF bunch, adiponectin expanded, leptin diminished (however this was not critical when standardized for fat mass), and T3 diminished fundamentally contrasted with ND, with no huge changes in TSH. No critical changes were discernible for lipids (complete cholesterol, HDL-c and LDL-c), with the exception of an abatement of TG in TRF bunch. TNF-and IL-1 beta were lower in TRF at the finish of the examination when contrasted with ND. A huge abatement of respiratory proportion in TRF bunch was recorded.

1.4 Discussion

Fasting is a generally very much contemplated metabolic state in sports and actual exercise because of investigations of the "Ramadan" period saw by Muslim competitors. Notwithstanding, just a solitary report has revealed its impact during an opposition preparing program pointed toward accomplishing skeletal muscle development. Our information exhibit that during a RT program, TRF was equipped for keeping up bulk, diminishing muscle versus fat, and decreasing aggravation markers. Be that as it may, it likewise diminished anabolic chemicals such testosterone and IGF-1.

A central issue of the TRF approach used in the current investigation is that all out every day calorie admission continued as before while the recurrence of dinners (for example time between dinners) was modified. This is not at all like numerous other IF regimens. There are various unique IF conventions, the majority of which have the objective of diminishing complete energy admission. Furthermore, dissimilar to ADF and some different types of IF, the routine used in the current investigation utilized a similar timetable every day, comprising of 16 hours fasting and 8 hours taking care of.

Despite the fact that IF has gotten a lot of consideration as of late, most of studies have explored the impacts of IF in overweight, stout or subjects. In any case, little is thought about the impacts of such dietary regimens in competitors, and all the more explicitly, in muscle heads or opposition prepared people. The current examination gives the first inside and out examination of IF in this populace of competitors. Except for decreased fatty oils, our outcomes don't affirm past research recommending a constructive outcome of IF on blood lipid profiles, in any case, it must be considered that our subjects were competitors. The size of decrease in fatty oils was likewise more modest than is commonly found in people who have raised fixations before IF.

As detailed, a decline of fat mass in people performing IF was noticed. Taking into account that the aggregate sum of kilocalories and the supplement dispersion were not fundamentally unique between the two gatherings, the instrument of more noteworthy fat misfortune in IF bunch can't just be clarified by changes in the amount or nature of diet, yet rather by the distinctive fleeting feast circulation. Numerous organic components have been upheld to clarify these impacts. One is the increment of adiponectin that collaborates with adenosine 5-monophosphate-enacted protein kinase (AMPK) and animates Peroxisome proliferator-initiated receptor gamma coactivator 1-alpha (PGC-1) protein articulation and mitochondrial biogenesis. Also, adiponectin acts in the cerebrum to expand energy use and cause weight reduction. It is eminent that in the current examination, the distinctions in adiponectin between bunches stayed in any event, when standardized comparative with muscle versus fat mass, though the huge abatement of leptin (that may be viewed as a troublesome factor for fat misfortune) was not, at this point critical when standardized for fat mass. Other theory is an upgraded thermogenic reaction to epinephrine or an expansion in REE after brief times of fasting, yet our primer information didn't uphold this point.

Curiously, in spite of the fact that decreases in the anabolic chemicals testosterone and IGF-1 were noticed, this didn't compare to any malicious body synthesis changes or bargains of strong strength over the span of the examination. It has been recently announced that men performing caloric limitation have lower testosterone than those devouring non-confined Western eating regimens, notwithstanding, the current analysis didn't limit calories in the IF bunch. In creature models, IF impacts the gonadal hub and testosterone fixation most likely through an abatement in leptin-intervened impacts, however it should be viewed as that subject on an each and every other day taking care of routine devour around 30–40 % less calories after some time contrasted with free taking care of creatures and that in our investigation, no distinctions in leptin focus were seen when standardized for fat mass. Likewise, the decrease of IGF-1 in the TRF bunch merits some conversation. A past report revealed no progressions in the GH/IGF-1 during Ramadan intermittent fasting. Despite the fact that it is conceivable that IF imitates caloric limitation through normal pathways (for example AMPK/ACC), ongoing information on people showed no impacts of caloric limitation on IGF-1. It is conceivable that the expansion of adiponectin and the diminishing of leptin could impact the IGF-1 focus, despite the fact that it is muddled how much changes in adipokines sway circling IGF-1 levels following weight reduction.

Past examinations have announced blended outcomes concerning the capacity to keep up fit weight during IF, yet by far most of these investigations forced calorie limitation and didn't use practice mediations. In our investigation, the supplement timing identified with instructional course was diverse between the two gatherings, and this could influence the anabolic reaction of the subjects despite the fact that these impacts are as yet hazy. Notwithstanding, we didn't track down any critical contrasts between bunches in without fat mass, demonstrating that the impact of supplement timing might be unimportant when the general substance of the eating regimen is comparable.

There is an expanding measure of information proposing that IF might actually be an achievable nourishing plan to battle certain infections. In the current investigation, both blood glucose and insulin fixations diminished in the

IF bunch. The capability of IF to balance blood glucose and insulin fixations has recently been talked about, however essentially with regards to overweight and hefty people. The simultaneous expansion in adiponectin and decline in insulin might be identified with regulation of insulin affectability, as adiponectin fixations have been emphatically related with insulin affectability. Besides, identified with the notable calming impact of adiponectin, it is conceivable that the decrease of incendiary markers is identified with the improvement of insulin affectability. Irritation assumes an urgent part in insulin opposition advancement through various cytokines that impact various atomic pathways. For instance, insulin obstruction could be set off by TNF pathways, which may expand serine/threonine phosphorylation of insulin receptor substrate 1. In addition IL-6 could diminish insulin affectability in skeletal muscle by actuating cost like receptor-4 (TLR-4) quality articulation through STAT3 (activator of record 3) enactment. This relationship is possibly bidirectional as the enactment of flagging could, thus, invigorate the creation of TNF. Adjustment of a portion of these fiery markers by IF was found in the current investigation: TNF and IL-1 beta were lower in the TRF bunch than ND at the finish of the examination, while IL-6 seemed to diminish in the TRF bunch, yet was not fundamentally not the same as ND. Past data on the effect of IF on provocative markers is restricted, yet a past examination detailed no progressions in TNF or IL-6 following fourteen days of altered IF in a little example of solid young fellows.

Albeit a decrease in T3 was seen in the IF bunch, no progressions in TSH or resting energy use were noticed. The noticed decrease in RR in the TRF bunch shows an exceptionally little shift towards dependence on unsaturated fats for fuel very still, albeit a critical factual association for RR was absent. Fasting RR has been recently answered to be an indicator of generous future weight acquire in non-corpulent men, with people who have higher fasting RR being bound to put on weight. Strangely, it was accounted for that in spite of the fact that RR was identified with future weight acquire, RMR was definitely not. It ought to be noticed that people with the most elevated danger of future weight acquire had fasting RR is equivalent to 0.85 (when contrasted with people who had RR is equivalent to 0.76). In the current investigation, the RR toward the finish of the examination in both the TRF gathering and ND bunch don't straightforwardly fall into both of these classes (RR is equivalent to 0.81 and 0.83 separately).

In view of the current investigation, an adjusted IF convention (for example TRF) could be doable for strength competitors without contrarily influencing strength and bulk. Curiously, despite the fact that androgen focuses were brought down by TRF, there was no distinction in bulk changes between gatherings. Caloric limitation in subject has been accounted for to diminish testosterone and IGF-1 despite the fact that human information on long haul serious caloric limitation doesn't show a decline in IGF-1 levels, yet rather an expanded serum insulin-like development factor restricting protein 1 (IGFBP-1) fixation. Nonetheless, no information are accessible for most types of IF. Abatement the action of the IGF-1 pivot could be an attractive objective for diminishing malignancy hazard, yet it is additionally notable that the initiation of the IGF-1/AKT (insulin-like development factor-1/protein kinase B/mammalian objective) pathway is one of the keys for strong development. As well as modifying IGF-1, fasting can advance autophagy, which is significant for ideal muscle wellbeing. Furthermore, there is a likelihood that the diverse eating examples of the gatherings in the current examination affected the general commitments of various hypertrophic pathways in each gathering.

A few constraints of the current examination ought to be considered. One is the distinctive planning of suppers in relationship to the instructional meetings that might have influenced the subjects' reactions. On this point, there isn't an agreement among analysts. The useful impacts of pre-practice fundamental amino corrosive starch supplement have been proposed, yet a similar gathering found that ingesting 20 g of whey protein either previously or 1 hour after 10 arrangements of leg augmentation brought about comparative paces of AA take-up. Also, different investigations have announced no advantage with pre-practice AA taking care of. Another impediment of the current investigation is that the energy and macronutrient structure of the eating regimen depended on meeting, and this methodology has known shortcomings. Due to the constraints of this strategy, it is conceivable that distinctions in energy or supplement consumption between gatherings might have existed and assumed a part in the noticed results.

Chapter 2. Impact of Intermittent Fasting on Resting Energy Expenditure

As of late, interest in time-confined taking care of (TRF) has expanded from reports featuring upgrades in body piece and solid execution measures. 26 casually dynamic guys were haphazardly doled out to one or the other TRF (n is equivalent to 13; 22.9 years; 82.0 kg; 178.1 cm; 8 hours eating window, 25% caloric shortfall, 1.8 g/kg/day protein) or typical eating routine (ND; n is equivalent to 13; 22.5 years; 83.3 kg; 177.5 cm; ordinary dinner design; 25% caloric deficiency, 1.8 g/kg/day protein) gatherings. Members went through about a month of regulated full body obstruction preparing. Changes in body piece (fat mass (FM), fat free mass (FFM), and muscle versus fat ratio (BF%)), skeletal muscle cross sectional territory (CSA) and muscle thickness (MT) of the vastus lateralis (VL), rectus femoris, (RF), and biceps brachii (BB) muscles, resting energy use (REE), strong execution, blood biomarkers, and psychometric boundaries were evaluated. Critical (p is equivalent to 0.05) diminishes were noted in BM, FM, BF%, testosterone, adiponectin, and REE, alongside huge expansions in the two gatherings. Plasma cortisol levels were altogether raised at post (p = 0.018) just in ND. Furthermore, FFM was kept up similarly between gatherings. Consequently, a TRF way of eating doesn't upgrade decreases in FM over caloric limitation alone during a 4-week hypo caloric eating regimen.

2.1 Introduction

Fasting can be characterized as restraint from ingesting food and caloric drinks for indicated time-frames, going from hours to a little while. As of late, fasting has developed from its very much reported roots in strict practices to a typical dietary procedure in both athletic and clinical fields, frequently for the objective of improving body creation or cardio metabolic wellbeing markers. As of now, there are a large number of fasting conventions sorted as intermittent fasting (IF) including substitute day fasting (ADF) and adjusted substitute day fasting, entire day fasting, and time-limited taking care of (TRF). While an extensive assessment of the contrasts between the different types of IF is past the extent of this report and it is imperative to feature a few shared characteristics. Every variation uses a characterized time of forbearance from all calories that broadens the overnight quick and frequently prompts decreases in generally speaking caloric admission, going from 25 to 38%. This has driven numerous to address whether changes in the physiological results (e.g., body piece and cardio metabolic wellbeing markers) regularly connected with fasting conventions are ascribed to the novel advantages of fasting itself, or exclusively because of the resultant caloric limitation. While past examinations have analyzed the likely effect of IF on body synthesis and metabolic wellbeing markers, most of examinations have been done in overweight and corpulent populaces and without the execution of an organized exercise program. Moreover, these examinations have basically utilized either ADF styles of fasting, rather than the more normally rehearsed TRF.

INTERMITTENT
FASTING

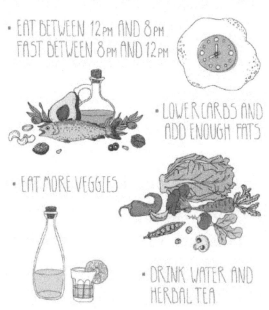

- EAT BETWEEN 12PM AND 8PM
  FAST BETWEEN 8PM AND 12PM
- LOWER CARBS AND
  ADD ENOUGH FATS
- EAT MORE VEGGIES
- DRINK WATER AND
  HERBAL TEA

TRF is customarily described as every day caloric forbearance going from 12 to 20 hours followed by not indispensable food and liquid utilization for the excess hours of the 24-hours' time frame. Tragically, there is a shortage of logical writing on this type of IF by and large and an especially perceptible absence of information in practicing populaces, among whom TRF is frequently drilled. Two regular TRF varieties include an everyday 16-hours quick with a 8-hours taking care of window (16/8; e.g., the Lean Gains Diet) or a day by day 20-hours quick with 4-hours taking care of window (20/4; e.g., the Warrior Diet). Until this point in time, just three past mediations have been completed in obstruction prepared populaces, two of which utilized the 16/8 convention, while the other analyzed a changed 20/4 routine. To begin with, the work is inspected fasting on exchanging days. In particular, beforehand undeveloped men were approached to follow a fasting convention for about two months comprising of 4-hours taking care of windows four days of the week, with not indispensable taking care of the leftover three days out of every week, on which they additionally opposition prepared. Overall, 667 kcals, 75 g of carbs, 25 g of fat, and 30 g of protein (comparing to 0.4 g/kg) less on fasting days than non-fasting days, no critical contrasts were noted for weight (BM), lean delicate tissue (LST), or fat mass (FM). Moreover, solid execution transformations were not restrained in the TRF bunch, with upgrades noted for both lower body strength and perseverance just as chest area strength toward the finish of the 8-week examination.

Comparable discoveries were accounted for by Moro and associates, who examined a 16/8 TRF convention in all around prepared men. Dissimilar to members in the TRF bunch were needed to quick ordinarily all through the span of the investigation rather than simply on non-preparing days. Besides, the two gatherings revealed burning-through generally a similar number of kcals (3000 kcals/day) and protein (2.0g/kg/day) spread out across three dinners. The non-fasting bunch burned-through their suppers at 8 am, 1 pm, and 8 pm, while the TRF bunch devoured their dinners at 1 pm, 4 pm, and 8 pm. Accordingly, all members went through directed preparing led threefold week by week, comprising of hefty compound developments to disappointment. Body organization, resting metabolic rate, basal degrees of anabolic and yearning chemicals, and solid execution were analyzed pre-and post-the 8-week intercession. The TRF bunch experienced critical reductions in FM, leptin, complete testosterone, adiponectin, IGF-1, and expansions in the adipokine adiponectin. Despite the fact that, it should be noticed that huge contrasts for leptin were not, at this point clear once adjusted for BM. Moreover, there were no huge contrasts found in fat free mass (FFM) or solid execution. At last, a comparative examination was done in obstruction prepared females by partners in 2019. 24 members went through about two months of regulated preparing while, similar as, following either a 16/8 fasting convention or having routinely from breakfast until the finish of day. Besides, all members burned-through a normal of 1.6g/kg/day of protein. In a for each convention investigation of 24 members who finished the mediation and conformed to contemplate systems, a critical gathering by time association demonstrated more noteworthy loss of FM in the TRF and TRF in addition to (HMB) supplementation bunches comparative with the typical eating regimen bunch at the 4-week time point, however the FM misfortune just remained genuinely huge for the TRF in addition to HMB bunch before the finish of the examination. Notwithstanding, no huge contrasts between bunches were seen in the goal to-treat investigation that incorporated every one of the 40 members who entered the examination. By and by, no distinction in changes in FFM were noted between gatherings, with all gatherings showing an increment. Additionally, all gatherings showed expanded muscle thickness of the elbow flexors and knee extensors just as solid execution upgrades without contrasts between gatherings. With the unique discoveries in FM changes between the three past examinations, and the generous premium in TRF projects to adjust body creation, further examination is required, utilizing a more powerful strategy for body piece appraisal (e.g., multi-compartment models contrasted with double energy X-beam absorptiometry). Moreover, because of the restricted writing in opposition preparing populaces, there is a requirement for additional investigation of whether TRF impacts transformations to obstruction preparing when calorie and protein admissions are controlled. Subsequently, the current examination looked to develop the work by further investigating the effect of transient TRF. All the more explicitly, noted huge enhancements in body arrangement at about a month in the TRF bunch, however these progressions not, at this point stayed at about two months. Along these lines, a month was picked for our examination to additionally clarify the expected impacts of more limited time spans of calorie prohibitive counting calories. Furthermore, 4-week caloric limitation time-frames may likewise be more delegate of field executions of TRF in sporting populaces (e.g., enhancements in body arrangement or weight while topping for strength sports). Moreover, because of the restricted exploration on obstruction preparing and TRF, this information couldn't just be recounting the more intense changes in body organization, strong execution, resting energy consumption, and blood biomarkers, yet be based upon by future examination contemplates that carry out a comparable plan for longer time-frames (e.g., 8–24 weeks). In this way, our goal was to examine the impacts of 16/8 TRF versus a typical dinner appropriation with identical calorie shortages and protein consumption in the two gatherings on proportions of body structure, strong execution, resting energy use, and blood biomarkers following a month of obstruction preparing in casually dynamic men.

2.2 Methods

Experimental Design

The current examination incorporated a sum of 16 visits (two pre-mediation research facility visits, 12 preparing visits, two post-intercession lab visits) over a 6-week time span. Preceding the initiation of testing, members were educated regarding the prerequisites of taking an interest in the investigation, evaluated and marked an institutional audit board (IRB)- endorsed assent structure showing their readiness to take part, and finished wellbeing history and hazard separation polls. Members were then arbitrarily appointed (i.e., basic randomization) to one of two gatherings: TRF with a 25% caloric shortfall or ordinary every day taking care of (ND) with a 25% caloric deficiency. All lab testing was led in the activity physiology lab, while all directed instructional meetings were held at the on location obstruction preparing office. The examination was endorsed by the college. All information were gathered as per the affirmation.

Participants

The ideal number of members for a two-way rehashed measures investigation of fluctuation was resolved through a force examination using an impact size of 0.3 and a force of 0.8 (nonexclusive info). It was resolved that an all-out example size of 24 would be required by means of the force examination. 32 guys between the ages of 18 and 35 years were enrolled for the examination to represent potential nonconformists or members who didn't hold fast to the examination rules. All members were sorted as casually dynamic, which was operationally characterized as taking part in obstruction preparing 2–4 times each week for as far back as a half year. Members were liberated from muscular wounds (inside the previous five years) just as cardiovascular, metabolic, and aspiratory messes that would contraindicate cooperation in the testing or preparing conventions associated with the investigation. All members had not gone through any critical weight reduction (10% of body weight) in a half year preceding enlistment and were not at present rehearsing any TRF conventions. People who had a past filled with dietary issues were rejected from cooperation. Moreover, any member utilizing anabolic steroids or at present taking drugs (e.g., steroidal and non-steroidal) or dietary enhancements (e.g., creatine, beta-alanine, fish oil) that might have meddled with the examination results were not selected.

2.3 Laboratory Assessment

Overview

During the underlying visit, members were approached to show up in active wear after an overnight quick (8 hours) and abstention from caffeine (12 hours) and demanding activity (24 hours). Members were given an outline of the investigation, given their composed agree to partake, and finished all clinical, exercise, and dietary surveys. All volunteers were then randomized into one of two gatherings, TRF or ND, and finished an appraisal of resting energy consumption (REE) by means of circuitous calorimeter. Following these techniques, members went through a blood draw for the assortment of serum and plasma, body creation appraisal by means of the 4-compartment (4C) model, ultrasonography for evaluation of muscle morphology, and vertical leap (VJ) acquaintance.

Visit 2 was finished 48–96 h following Visit 1 and comprised of proportions of activity execution including VJ, leg press one-reiteration most extreme, seat press one-redundancy greatest, leg press redundancies to disappointment with a heap comparing to 65%, and seat press reiterations to disappointment with a heap relating to 65%. Endless supply of all benchmark information assortment, members went through four sequential long stretches of an occasional obstruction preparing program comprising of multiple times week after week full body schedules in an everyday undulating periodization plot with both pre-intercession visits continued after preparing culmination. Every member's post-trying visit time happened inside 2 hours of the pre-testing visit time. Visit 15 happened 72–96 hours after the last instructional meeting. Visit 16 was the last visit, happening 48–96 hours after Visit 15.

Anthropometric Measurements

Weight was estimated toward the start of each body arrangement preliminary utilizing an aligned scale. Members wore just pressure shorts and a dip cap during weight appraisals. Stature was estimated following enlistment into the examination during the main visit. All tallness estimations were finished utilizing a similar adjusted meter.

Body Composition

During pre-and post-intercession appraisals, a 4C model was used to evaluate body organization. This model required evaluations by means of double energy X-beam absorptiometry, air uprooting diagram, and bioelectrical impedance investigation. All bits of hardware were aligned the morning of every appraisal as per the producer's rules. DXA, ADP, and BIA gave appraisals of bone mineral substance, absolute body volume, and all out body water, individually. These factors were gone into the 4C condition to decide FM, FFM, and muscle versus fat ratio for every member.

Ultrasound

Muscle morphology (cross-sectional territory (CSA), muscle thickness (MT), and muscle quality (reverberation force (EI)) was assessed utilizing ultrasound with a 12-MHz straight test checking head for the accompanying musculature: m. rectus femoris (RF), m. vastus lateralis (VL), and m. biceps brachii (BB). All pictures were taken by a similar expert, who had recently illustrated "great" unwavering quality in a populace of school matured guys and females. Going before all evaluations, a standard profundity and gain was set. To guarantee that the test moved along a cross over plane of the muscle, froth cushioning was taped to the skin opposite to the longitudinal pivot of the ideal site. Three pictures were gathered at each site. Subcutaneous fat thickness for the two muscles was estimated utilizing the straight line capacity and used to ascertain standardized EI. The normal of the nearest two pictures were hence utilized for examination. All pictures were moved to a PC for examination through Image. CSA was resolved utilizing the polygon work in Image to choose however much of the objective muscle as could be expected with no encompassing bone or belt. The distance between the shallow aponeurosis to the profound aponeurosis was utilized to decide muscle thickness. Muscle quality was resolved from the reverberation power esteems evaluated from a similar locale as CSA. The mean reverberation power esteem was determined as a dim scale esteem between 0 (dark) and 255 (white) subjective units. Explicit destinations for ultrasound were gathered as recently depicted: (1) RF at half of the longitudinal distance of the foremost prevalent iliac spine and the predominant line of the patella (5 cm profundity; 50 addition); (2) VL at half of the longitudinal distance of the more noteworthy trochanter to the sidelong epicondyle of the femur while keeping a 10 knee point (5 cm profundity; 50 increase); and (3) BB at 66% of the separation from the average acromion cycle to the cubital fossa while lying in a prostrate situation with shoulder kidnapped (4 cm profundity; 58 increase).

Resting Energy Expenditure

REE was surveyed through aberrant calorimeter. Gas and stream alignments were played out every early daytime as per the producer's details, and the pre-evaluation methods of were used. Volunteers laid prostrate in a dull space for 20–30 minutes with a ventilated hood set over their face and neck. REE was resolved dependent on a 5-min timespan volume of oxygen utilization (VO2) with a coefficient of variety (CV) 5%.

Analysis of Blood

The member's abstained blood tests were acquired pre- and post-mediation. Blood tests were acquired from a vein by an examination colleague who was prepared in phlebotomy. Around 20 mL of blood was brought into serum-isolating (SST) (for serum assortment) and (EDTA)- treated cylinders (for plasma). SST tubes were permitted to clump for 10 min preceding centrifugation, while EDTA treated cylinders were tenderly reversed and centrifuged. Tests were centrifuged for 10 min at 3600 rpm at 4 °C. The subsequent serum and plasma were aliquot and put away at less 80 °C until investigation.

Plasma cortisol, serum testosterone, serum adiponectin, leptin, and absolute ghrelin were totally dissected in copy by means of protein connected immunsorbent examines (ELISA). All ELISA packs were perused utilizing per user, as per the unit rules. The between examine coefficient of varieties (CV) and qualities for everything biomarkers can be found.

Vertical Jump

Vertical leap tallness (VJHT) and pinnacle power (VJPP) information were gathered utilizing a convenient power plate testing at 1000 Hz. Three maximal counter development bounces (CMJ) were performed with one moment of rest between endeavors. All CMJ were completed with the members setting their hands on their hips and quickly diving to a self-chose profundity before bouncing with maximal exertion. The members were told to try not to play out a fold bounce. VJHT and VJPP were totally evaluated during the concentric period of the CMJ. Information were dissected by means of programming.

Estimated One Repetition Maximum

Assessed one reiteration maximums were resolved for the hand weight seat press and leg press works out. For the two activities, members were approached to finish a particular warm-up, as recently depicted, comprising of five redundancies with 20% of the assessed 1RM, trailed by three reiterations at half of the assessed 1RM, two reiterations at 75% 1RM, lastly one reiteration at 85% of their assessed 1RM. In this manner, sets of five redundancies were finished with expanding weight until the member could not, at this point total the set, with 5 min of rest between maximal endeavors. All maximal endeavor loads were chosen by the specialist dependent on the reiterations for possible later use announced by the member toward the fulfillment of each set and visual bar speed all through each endeavor. Every member's sub 5RM was resolved inside three to five endeavors. When every member's sub 5RM was accomplished, results were gone into the 1RM assessment equation for the last assurance of e1RM. The seat press was performed with the member's favored grasp width and the necessity that the bar connected with the chest and got back to the beginning position. A redundancy was just considered 'acceptable' (i.e., checked) if the member finished the reiteration with feet on the floor and hips and upper back excess in contact with the seat. For a leg press endeavor to be viewed as fruitful, the member's legs were needed to plummet to a 90° point between the lower leg and thigh, at that point get back to the beginning position while the remainder of the body stayed in contact with the seat. Preceding all leg press sets, foot position was estimated to guarantee all maximal endeavors were finished in a similar way. All sets were finished with prepared spotters from the examination group to guarantee legitimate strategy and wellbeing, all things considered.

Muscular Endurance

Five minutes after leg press and seat press e1RM had been set up, strong perseverance was resolved using 65% e1RM for a solitary set until solid disappointment for the two activities. The request for practice performed was equivalent to 1RM testing (i.e., seat press followed by leg press). Disappointment was characterized as the main reiteration that necessary help from a spotter, or in which a breakdown in strategy was seen during the redundancy. All endeavors were performed with a similar hand and foot situation as the 1RM testing and under the management of individuals from the exploration group to guarantee the security of the member.

Questionnaires

The apparent recuperation scale (PRS) was finished upon appearance to each instructional course, while the everyday examinations of life requests for competitors (DALDA) and visual simple scales (VAS) for energy, want to eat, craving, totality, and inspiration to do actual assignments were finished upon appearance to the primary instructional course of every week all through the examination. Moreover, the DALDA and three-factor eating poll were finished during pre-and post-testing body organization visits, preceding ultrasound assessment. The PRS was evaluated on a 0–10 scale with

0 addressing 'inadequately recuperated/incredibly drained' and 10 addressing 'all around recuperated/exceptionally vigorous'. The VAS were additionally surveyed on a scale going from 0 to 10 (0 methods no energy, no craving to eat, no yearning, not full, no inspiration and 10 is incredibly vigorous, outrageous longing to eat, very eager, amazingly full, incredibly propelled). The DALDA comprises of two sections (A and B) and contains a joined all out of 34 inquiries decided on a 3-point scale (a methods more regrettable than typical, b is equivalent to ordinary, c is equivalent to better than ordinary). It contains 17 inquiries dependent on a 4-point scale (1 is certainly bogus, 2 is equivalent to for the most part bogus, 3 is generally obvious, 4 is unquestionably evident) and one inquiry scored 1 to 8 on eating limitation (1 is equivalent to no restriction when eating, 8 is outrageous restriction when eating). It at that point gives scores to intellectual limitation, enthusiastic eating, and uncontrolled eating between 0–100.

2.4 Intervention

Dietary Program

Randomization into one of two gatherings happened: (1) TRF: time-limited taking care of with all calorie and macronutrient utilization happening inside a 8 hours duration every day and a recommended 25% caloric shortage; and (2) ND: ordinary day by day taking care of timetable with an endorsed 25% caloric deficiency.

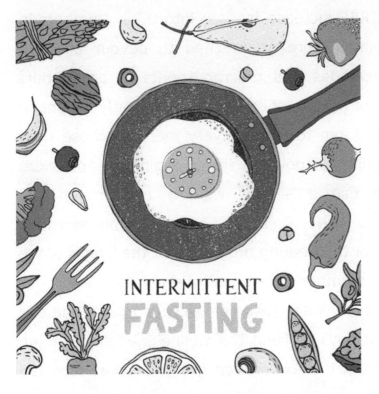

Notwithstanding the 25% caloric limitation endorsed to the two gatherings, all members were approached to devour 1.8 g/kg/day of dietary protein to advance ideal FFM variations. Furthermore, on preparing days 50g of hydrolyzed whey protein detach was given to all members upon the finish of every exercise to guarantee ideal post exercise supplement timing. The excess calories were scattered among carb and fat admission at the carefulness of the member. Upkeep calories were assessed as REE increased by a standard movement factor of 1.5. In this way, the last condition for recommended every day calories was as per the following: (REE increase by 1.5) into 0.75. Members in the TRF bunch were approached to devour all their necessary calories and macronutrients in an 8-hours taking care of window of one or the other early afternoon to 8 pm or 1 pm to 9 pm. Every member chose their favored eating window at study beginning and were needed to use a similar window all through the examination. The ND bunch had no time sensitive limitations for their eating program. For the length of the mediation, member's revealed dietary admission for three days every week (two non-weekend days, one end of the week day) utilizing the wellness application. An individual from the exploration group checked food log consistence every week during obstruction instructional meetings. All out calories, relative calories, sugar (grams), fat (grams), and protein (grams) were gathered from food logs. Normal macronutrient and calorie admissions were thought about between gatherings.

Resistance Training Protocol

The 4-week preparing convention comprised of full body meetings performed three times each week. The leg press and seat press were acted in all meetings, trailed by a flat paddling exercise, a shoulder exercise, quadriceps and hamstring predominant activities acted in really set design, and rear arm muscles and bicep practices proceeded as a superset. The seat press practice was performed with two minutes of rest between sets, though the rest stretch between all single leg press and flat paddling practices was 90 s. At last, all shoulder and very set activities were isolated by one moment of rest. The exercises continued in a day by day undulating periodization design with seat and leg press redundancies going from 3 to 8. The seat press loads depended on rates from the pre-mediation e1RM. All resulting practices were performed to a recommended scope of reiterations available for later. All instructional courses were directed under analyst watch. Members were needed to check in toward the start of all instructional meetings and complete the meeting as recommended to be considered consistent with the preparation convention. Instructional meetings happened in the early evening between 3 pm and 8 pm, during the members' taking care of window. Members who had not exactly a 90% consistence rate were prohibited from the investigation.

Statistical Analysis

The suspicion of ordinariness was affirmed with the test (p is equivalent to 0.05). Free examples t-test were utilized to survey gauge contrasts between gatherings. Subordinate factors were broke down utilizing two-way (bunch increase by time) rehashed measures investigations of difference (ANOVA). In case of a critical association, the POST time point was thought about between bunches utilizing a free examples t-test with change. Incomplete estimated time of arrival squared impact sizes were determined for investigations of difference discoveries, though Cohen's d impact sizes were resolved for the t-test results. A rule alpha degree of p is equivalent to 0.05 was utilized to decide factual importance. Information were broke down utilizing the measurable bundle SPSS. All information were introduced as mean SD (except if in any case noted).

2.5 Results

Participants

32 members were enlisted to take an interest in the examination, while 30 members finished the investigation. Of the two members who neglected to finish the investigation, one intentionally eliminated himself for individual reasons, while the second neglected to stick to post-testing timing methods. Both of these members were in the ND bunch. From the 30 members that finished the examination, 26 were remembered for the last investigation. One individual was prohibited for absence of adherence to the fasting convention (TRF gathering), and three were barred for absence of dietary adherence (i.e., rebelliousness with appointed macronutrient or kcal utilization) by means of dietary logs gathered all through the examination. The autonomous examples t-tests showed no huge contrasts between bunches for pattern upsides of every single ward variable. Member qualities for the last 26 members remembered for the investigation are shown.

Dietary Intake

No critical contrasts were noted between bunches for admissions of 4-week normal protein, carb, fat, all out calories, or calories per kilogram of bodyweight all through the examination

Muscular Performance

Fundamental impacts for time were noted for (p is equivalent to 0.001), albeit no gathering into time communications were seen for one or the other variable. Besides, no primary impacts for time or gathering into time collaborations were noted for all things considered.

Psychometric Parameters

Principle impacts for time were seen for intellectual limitation. No fundamental impacts for time or gathering into time associations were noted for enthusiastic eating, uncontrolled eating, seen recuperation between instructional meetings, VAS (energy, want to eat, completion, yearning, and inspiration to do actual assignments), or view of day by day life stressors.

Blood Biomarkers

A principle impact for time was noticed for testosterone, leptin, and adiponectin, demonstrating a diminishing in all members joined. Notwithstanding, no critical gathering into time associations were noted. A gathering into time communication was noted for cortisol. Post hoc free examples t-tests uncovered no distinctions in cortisol fixations among ND and TRF at standard (p is equivalent to 0.652), however higher focuses in ND when contrasted with TRF at post (p is equivalent to 0.018). The between measure coefficient of varieties (CV) and qualities for everything biomarkers can be seen.

2.6 Discussion

As of late, fasting regimens, for example, TRF have acquired significant fame in spite of restricted exact help for their benefits when contrasted with conventional energy-limited weight control plans. The current investigation exhibited transient TRF didn't evoke more ideal modifications in body structure when contrasted with an ordinary feast circulation in isocaloric and isonitrogenous conditions. In any case, our information additionally propose that 16/8 TRF doesn't adversely impact the capacity to keep up FFM more than about a month in a hypo caloric state when raised dietary protein admission and an exhausting obstruction preparing program are available. Also, the execution of everyday 16-hours fasting periods didn't bargain enhancements in solid strength or control throughout the span of the mediation.

While the current investigation was more limited than the three past TRF and opposition preparing mediations (i.e., four instead of about two months, generally comparative body synthesis changes were as yet noted. Tinsley and associates noted clear contrasts in LST changes among fasting and non-fasting bunches throughout the span of about two months, which, albeit not measurably huge, may have pragmatic ramifications for those performing opposition preparing for body synthesis improvement. The scientists hypothesized that these variations may be ascribed to the varying normal day by day protein admissions between the gatherings. Notwithstanding, regardless of the lower protein consumption, LST was kept up with TRF, probably because of the opposition preparing improvement. While trying to take out inconsistencies in protein admission, Moro and partners and coordinated with protein between bunches at 1.9 g/kg/day and 1.6 g/kg/day, individually. Following two months of 16/8 TRF in opposition prepared guys, it is accounted for FFM was kept up, loaning belief to detailed speculation that protein admission was the reasonable wellspring of the potential errors in lean mass changes in their past examination. Furthermore, Tinsley et al. (2019) announced expansions in FFM paying little heed to bunch (i.e., TRF, TRF in addition to HMB, control), regardless of contrasts in feast timing. Hence, the current investigation also upholds the three past mediations, without any distinctions in the support of FFM between gatherings, regardless of contrasts in dinner timing and the resultant disparities in every day energy and protein conveyance. With the execution of a 25% caloric shortfall, huge declines in BM credited to loss of both FM and FFM would be normal without an organized exercise program and sufficient protein admission. As the two gatherings comparably diminished BM, FM, and BF% following the 4-week intercession, and FFM didn't transform, it very well may be derived that the activity and nourishment mediation was compelling for advancing loss of muscle to fat ratio without simultaneous fit mass misfortune. Past research recommends that a protein admission of 2 g/kg/day might be needed to keep up FFM during an energy-limited eating routine in dynamic people as protein is basic for up directing muscle protein blend, the main thrust behind FFM versatile reactions to ongoing obstruction work out. While our members were not burning-through 2 g/kg/day, they without a doubt devoured 1.8 g/kg/d, an amount outperforming the 1.6 g/kg/d limit featured by Morton and partners for expanding bulk while participating in obstruction preparing just as in the proposed scope of 1.4–2.0 g/kg/day suggested by the International Society of Sports Nutrition. It is conceivable the multi day out of every week, full body obstruction practice program, alongside a higher protein diet, added to these outcomes.

REE diminished correspondingly for the two gatherings following the 4-week mediation, be that as it may, this is in accordance with past discoveries. A methodical audit of 90 examinations showed a normal of 15.4 kcals/kg of weight reduction bringing down of REE. Curiously, the normal decrement was more prominent in intercessions enduring two to about a month and a half. The easing back of metabolic rate with weight reduction is frequently ascribed to decreases in FFM. In any case, as our members looked after FFM, this isn't probably going to be a contributing element to the decrease in REE saw in the current examination.

One of the significant errors between the current discoveries and Moro et al. is that of decreases in FM with the execution of TRF. Not at all like, had this examination exhibited that when every day caloric admission was compared, the changes in dinner recurrence didn't assume a part in the decreases of FM or BF%. These discoveries affirmed our theory that in general caloric equilibrium would be the driving element in changes in body piece, notwithstanding adjustments in dinner timing. In any case, the contrasting lengths and member attributes, especially preparing status, between these two investigations are critical. Furthermore, as the two examinations utilized self-announced dietary appraisals, the detailed healthful admissions ought to be seen carefully.

Members in the current examination expanded BP1RM and LP1RM to a huge degree, in spite of the fact that enhancements didn't contrast between eats less. While members didn't expand entire body FFM to a huge degree, results from muscle ultrasonography exhibited huge expansions in VL and BB CSA. It is conceivable that the improvement in both lower body and chest area strength measures throughout a brief timeframe can be halfway ascribed to expansions in CSA. While the CSA increments are eminent, past reports feature that a solid connection between expansions in CSA and strong strength are not grounded until tip top degrees of preparing status and capability have been accomplished. Given the short preparing span in the current examination, almost certainly, significant neural transformations were invigorated in light of the extreme obstruction preparing program executed in casually prepared members, and that these variations may have essentially added to the noticed strength increments. All things considered, the expansions in solid strength were like results announced by the past investigations around here. While solid strength improved, strong perseverance didn't improve for one or the other gathering in our examination. This is not normal for Tinsley and associates, who announced solid perseverance upgrades in the lower body. The absence of enhancements in strong perseverance in our examination are likely because of the way of preparing, instead of the dietary systems included.

Another opposite finding from the past examination was with respect to the biomarkers serum testosterone and plasma cortisol. Moro and partners announced declines in testosterone in the TRF bunch throughout about two months. Alternately, we tracked down no huge contrasts between bunches anytime all through the examination as to serum testosterone. While the brief time frame time of the current examination (a month) may have assumed a part in these discoveries, past examinations have discovered detectible changes in just one to about fourteen days of opposition preparing. It is significant that while we recognized a primary impact for time concerning diminishes in testosterone, the real physiological pertinence of noticed abatements is exceptionally sketchy as serum testosterone levels have been appeared to vacillate as much as 43% all through a 24 hours duration. Moreover, changes in rest examples may upset serum testosterone levels by as much as 57 ng/dl. In this manner, the minor adjustments noticed are likely not physiologically pertinent, in spite of factual importance, and ought not to be over-deciphered.

Also, our discoveries showed an ascent in plasma cortisol just in the ND bunch throughout about a month. Ascends in cortisol have been appeared to happen during hypo caloric periods, with more noteworthy builds discovered when members were asked to intently screen their weight control plans. Also, fasting has exhibited a capacity to change the ordinary circadian beat of cortisol rises and falls. While theoretical, the time of TRF may have modified the ordinary spike seen at the hour of day when cortisol was surveyed. While cortisol evaluations were taken at a similar surmised time pre-and post-mediation (2 hours), time from the waking hour was not measured, which may have likewise influenced the estimation. In any case, the past examination of Tinsley et al. shown no adjustment of the cortisol arousing reaction or changes in normal cortisol fixations with about two months of TRF in addition to opposition preparing in females. Future examinations ought to investigate the ramifications of TRF on cortisol levels and rhythms further. Also, the inconsistencies between the current examination's discoveries and that of partners (i.e., no adjustment of cortisol) may be inferable from the execution of a weight-upkeep diet, instead of an energy-confined eating routine.

One of the novel discoveries of the current examination was the absence of effect of TRF on saw competitor availability. In spite of the length of day by day calorie restraint, seen recuperation between instructional meetings and saw preparation didn't vary between abstains from food. This perspective has not been recently tended to as to TRF in obstruction preparing populaces, and might be helpful when choosing to execute TRF in effectively preparing people. Besides, the dietary methodology didn't fundamentally affect sensations of energy, inspiration to perform actual undertakings, totality, and want to eat, or hunger. Notwithstanding, feature that the circumstance of the reviews may have affected these discoveries as they were finished preceding the members' exercises, which fell inside their taking care of window.

There were various limits to the current investigation that ought not to be disregarded when deciphering the discoveries. To start with, the utilization of self-detailed dietary admission and putting together our dietary examination with respect to a sum of 12 days all through a month are constraints. Nonetheless, endeavors were made by the exploration group to guarantee members were holding fast to all dietary rules including talking with members during every exercise (i.e., three times each week) and investigating dietary logs toward the start of every week. We likewise perceive that the 4-week term of the investigation is a constraint and more examination should be led that executes longer time periods (e.g., 8–24 weeks). Besides, our members' circadian timetables, rest timetables, and work/scholarly timetables shifted, which may likewise impact our discoveries, particularly chemical evaluations. Also, we just inspected casually dynamic men. Future examinations ought to investigate assorted populaces and different levels of preparing status including applications to wear explicit execution. Also, variations of TRF design ought to be investigated, for example, utilizing TRF on work days with gets back to ordinary supper designs on ends of the week. Moreover, future examinations ought to look at the effect of exercise timing (i.e., preparing performed during or outside the taking care of window) on possible execution and body creation results related to TRF.

Conclusion

Indeed, even a solitary fasting span in people (e.g., overnight) can lessen basal convergences of numerous metabolic biomarkers related with persistent illness, like insulin and glucose. For instance, patients are needed to quick for 8–12 hours before blood attracts to accomplish consistent state fasting levels for some metabolic substrates and chemicals. A significant clinical and logical inquiry is whether receiving a standard, intermittent fasting routine is a plausible and economical populace based methodology for advancing metabolic wellbeing. Further, appropriately fueled, controlled clinical exploration is expected to test whether intermittent fasting regimens can supplement or supplant energy limitation and, provided that this is true, regardless of whether they can work with long haul metabolic enhancements and body weight the executives. The Summary Points are upheld by the current proof.

Also, intermittent fasting regimens endeavor to interpret the beneficial outcomes of fasting regimens in subject and different warm blooded creatures into commonsense eating designs for lessening the danger of constant sickness in people. In the Future Issues area, we propose issues that ought to be tended to in research examining intermittent fasting and metabolic wellbeing.

Lightning Source UK Ltd.
Milton Keynes UK
UKHW022014250521
384380UK00002B/187